Simplified Solution Approach

To INTERSTITIAL

CYSTITIS

Discover Healing Paths: A Comprehensive Guide to Reclaiming Your Wellness and Embracing Life's Vibrancy

Dr QUENTIN GLYN

Table Of Contents

CHAPTER ONE
Interstitial Cystitis

Urinary symptoms and bladder discomfort are the hallmarks of Interstitial Cystitis (IC), sometimes referred to as painful bladder syndrome. Its treatment often necessitates a multidisciplinary approach and has a substantial negative influence on the afflicted people's quality of life. The definition, prevalence, effect, and significance of early detection of infection control (IC) will all be covered in this approach to a simple solution.

Synopsis And Definition:

Urinary urgency, pain, and discomfort are symptoms of a persistent inflammatory illness of the bladder lining known as interstitial cystitis. Since IC doesn't react to traditional medications like bacterial illnesses do, diagnosing and treating it might be more difficult. Although the precise origin of IC is yet unknown, a complex interaction of immunological, genetic, and environmental variables is thought to be involved.

Numerous symptoms, including urgency, frequent urination, pelvic discomfort, and, in extreme situations, nocturia (regular nighttime urine), are often associated with IC. Individual differences exist in the intensity of symptoms, and the illness may have a major influence on relationships, everyday life, and mental health.

Frequency And Effects:

IC is more common than previously believed, impacting millions of people globally. Although it is more frequent in women, males may still have it. Many people with IC have pain and discomfort that interferes with their everyday activities, employment, and social relationships, which has a significant negative influence on their quality of life. Because IC is a chronic condition, mental anguish, anxiety, and depression may result.

The Value Of Early Identification

For better results and efficient care, early diagnosis of IC is essential. However, since the symptoms of IC may mimic those of other gynecological and urological disorders, identifying it can be difficult. When patients describe symptoms like frequent urination, urgency, or chronic pelvic discomfort, healthcare professionals need to pay close attention to them.

Stopping The Advancement And Complications:

Early detection of IC facilitates timely intervention and may stop the disease's development. If the illness is not addressed, it may lead to consequences including reduced bladder capacity and injury.

Increasing Life Quality:

People with IC have a higher quality of life as a result of improved symptom management brought about by early identification and care. Early in the course of the condition, patients may benefit from effective treatment techniques that include medication, physical therapy, and lifestyle adjustments that can help them better deal with their symptoms.

Conclusively, comprehending and managing Interstitial Cystitis necessitates an all-encompassing strategy that acknowledges the illness's description, frequency, consequences, and the significance of prompt identification. Healthcare professionals and people may both contribute to the improvement of the general health of persons afflicted with this chronic illness by being aware of the symptoms and indicators of IC and pushing for prompt diagnosis and treatment.

CHAPTER TWO
Cracking The Code

Urinary urgency and discomfort in the bladder are the hallmarks of Interstitial Cystitis (IC), sometimes referred to as painful bladder syndrome. Even though IC is a prevalent urological condition, its precise origin is still unknown. Investigating a range of variables, such as genetic, environmental, and autoimmune links, is necessary to unravel the riddle of IC.

Genetic Elements:

Familial Clustering: Studies point to a possible hereditary basis for IC. There is evidence of familial clustering, which suggests that those who have a family history of IC are more susceptible to the illness. This suggests that some people may be predisposed to IC due to hereditary causes.

Genetic Markers: Researchers are now looking at certain genetic markers linked to IC. Finding these markers may shed light on the condition's underlying processes. Research has investigated polymorphisms in genes associated with nerve function, bladder integrity, and inflammation as possible factors.

Environmental Stressors:

Toxic Exposures: Circumstances may either cause or worsen symptoms of IC. It has been studied how exposure to certain toxins, such as those found in personal care products or environmental contaminants, affects health. These chemicals may irritate the lining of the bladder, causing discomfort and inflammation.

Dietary Factors: One of the main causes of IC is diet. Caffeine, spicy meals, and acidic drinks are a few examples of foods and drinks that might exacerbate symptoms. One of the most important aspects of treating IC is recognizing and avoiding these triggers. Keeping up an inflammatory-reduction diet may also assist with symptoms.

Trauma and Infections: In some situations, pelvic trauma or prior UTIs may have a role in the development of IC. Chronic bladder pain may be brought on by chronic inflammation from untreated infections or accidents.

Autoimmune Relationships:

Immune System Dysfunction: Research on the immune system's involvement in IC is still in progress. According to some views, the bladder may be the focus of an aberrant immunological response, resulting in discomfort and inflammation. The body may unintentionally attack its own cells in the bladder wall via autoimmune processes.

Overlap with Other Autoimmune Conditions: Rheumatoid arthritis and lupus are two autoimmune diseases that often occur with inflammatory constipation (IC). This implies that immunological dysfunction and IC may be related. Both illnesses may emerge as a result of genetic vulnerability or shared immune mechanisms.

Inflammatory Mediators: Urine from people with IC has been shown to have higher concentrations of a few inflammatory mediators, including cytokines. This lends credence to the theory that an immune-mediated inflammatory response plays a role in the pathogenesis of IC.

In conclusion, a thorough investigation of genetic, environmental, and autoimmune variables is necessary to solve the puzzle of interstitial cystitis. Gaining insight into how these components interact might lead to more focused and efficient methods of diagnosing and treating this complex and sometimes crippling disease.

With further study, the complex processes causing IC are becoming clear, offering promise for better treatment and a higher standard of living for those who are afflicted.

CHAPTER THREE

Identifying Symptoms

Recognizing Indication:

1. Urination that hurts:

• Dysuria, or painful or unpleasant urinating, is one of the main signs and symptoms of IC.

• Burning or uncomfortable feelings may occur for those who have IC both during and after urinating.

• Pain may range in intensity from minor to severe, and it can also be intermittent or persistent.

2. Urgency and Frequency:

IC is often accompanied by an increased frequency of urine. This entails having to urinate more often than normal.

• Urgency to pee is also common; people may have a strong, overwhelming need to urinate right away.

• Only small quantities of pee may flow despite the urgency, which adds to the agony and aggravation that come with having IC.

3. Pelvic Pain:

• Pelvic pain, which may vary from a dull aching to excruciating anguish, is often brought on by IC.

• The discomfort might originate in the bladder region or spread to the perineum, lower back, and lower abdomen.

• Individuals with IC may experience discomfort that varies in severity and location.

4. Uneasiness during Sexual Activity:

• Pain or discomfort during sexual activity may be experienced by some persons with IC.

• A person's general quality of life and close relationships may be greatly impacted by this.

5. Nocturia:

• Nocturia is the term used to describe the need to urinate throughout the night.

• Nocturia is a common occurrence in people with IC, which throws off their sleep schedule and makes them tired.

Recognizing Typical Interstitial Cystitis Symptoms:

1. Exacerbations:

• The course of IC symptoms might change over time, with remission intervals interspersed with exacerbations of symptoms.

• Recognizing what foods, stress levels, or hormone fluctuations cause flare-ups is essential to controlling the illness.

2. Hematuria, or blood in the urine:

• During flare-ups, some IC patients may observe blood in their urine.

• If you have hematuria, it's crucial to speak with a healthcare provider since this may be a disturbing sign.

3. Urinary Bladder Wall Pain:

• Diagnostic tests, such as cystoscopy, may show redness (erythema) and small, pinpoint bleeding (glomerulations), which are indications of irritation of the bladder wall.

4. Effect on Life Quality:

• A person's general quality of life might be greatly impacted by IC.

The difficulties in controlling symptoms of chronic pain may lead to mental discomfort, worry, and depression in affected individuals.

5. Related Conditions:

• In addition to IC, some people may also suffer from fibromyalgia, chronic fatigue syndrome, or irritable bowel syndrome (IBS).

In summary, early diagnosis and successful treatment of Interstitial Cystitis depend on the ability to recognize symptoms and common indicators of the condition. Seeking medical attention is advised if a person has chronic urinary symptoms or believes they may have IC. A medical practitioner may do a comprehensive assessment, which includes a patient's medical history, physical examination, and diagnostic testing, to ascertain the best course of action for each patient.

CHAPTER FOUR

Uncovering Diagnosis Myths

The complicated and varied symptoms of Interstitial Cystitis (IC), a chronic inflammatory illness of the bladder, may make diagnosis difficult. Healthcare providers use a multimodal strategy that includes a patient's medical history, physical examination, and diagnostic testing in order to solve this puzzle and clear the path for an appropriate diagnosis. To comprehend the streamlined solution strategy for diagnosing interstitial cystitis, let's examine each component in more detail.

How To Handle The Diagnostic Procedure:

Health Background:

Symptom Assessment: It's critical to comprehend the patient's perspective. Symptoms of IC include urgency, frequency, nocturia, and pelvic discomfort. It is crucial to thoroughly examine these symptoms, their duration, and any aggravating or mitigating circumstances.

Voiding Patterns: Finding information about a person's voiding habits, such as how much fluid they consume, how often they void, and any patterns associated with food or drink, may assist in identifying possible triggers.

Medical and Medication History: Details on previous illnesses, surgeries, and prescription drugs are essential. Medications or health issues that are related to IC may exacerbate its symptoms.

Physical Assessment:

Pelvic Examination: A targeted pelvic examination helps to detect any abnormalities or soreness in the pelvic area. Specific pelvic floor muscles may be palpated to detect trigger points or muscle spasms related to IC.

Neurological Examination: Reflexes and sensory function assessments may provide more information since IC may have neurological ramifications.

Diagnostic Procedures And Tests:

Urine Analysis: Regular urine analysis may reveal indicators of inflammation and aid in the ruling out of UTIs. Elevated potassium levels, for example, might be a sign of bladder discomfort.

Cystoscopy: The gold standard diagnostic method, cystoscopy allows for direct sight of the bladder. It enables the medical professional to see ulcers, Hunner's lesions, or other symptoms of inflammation that are typical with IC.

Urodynamic Studies: These examinations evaluate the function of the bladder and may be used to spot irregularities in the flow and pressure of urine during voiding. Important information on bladder capacity and detrusor muscle function may be obtained from urodynamic investigations.

Potassium Sensitivity Test (PST): During a cystoscopy, potassium chloride is injected into the bladder. The patient's reaction is monitored to determine whether or not IC is present. During the exam, people with IC may feel more pain or discomfort.

Healthcare practitioners may create a thorough diagnosis of Interstitial Cystitis by combining the data from the physical examination, medical history, and diagnostic procedures. This all-encompassing method guarantees that the distinctive features of the patient's experience are taken into consideration, as well as any possible confounding variables. Initiating effective treatment methods and enhancing the quality of life for patients with IC need a timely and correct diagnosis.

CHAPTER FIVE

Options For Treatment

Urinary urgency and discomfort in the bladder are the hallmarks of interstitial cystitis (IC), sometimes referred to as painful bladder syndrome. A multifaceted strategy is used to manage interstitial cystitis, integrating several therapy modalities to reduce symptoms and enhance the patient's quality of life. A thorough summary of the available treatments is provided below:

1. Integrative Methods For Treating Interstitial Cystitis:

The goal of holistic treatments is to treat the patient's whole health, taking into account lifestyle, emotional, and physical aspects.

• Modifications to Diet:

• Steering clear of some meals and drinks, such as those high in acidity, caffeine, artificial sweeteners, and spices, since these may cause irritation to the bladder.

• It might be helpful to include meals that are favorable to the bladder, such as those that are low in acid and non-irritating.

• Managing Stress:

• IC symptoms may become worse under stress. Deep breathing exercises, mindfulness, and meditation are examples of stress-reduction strategies that may help control symptoms.

• Manual Therapy:

• Pelvic floor physical therapy is a useful treatment for bladder function improvement and pelvic floor muscle stress.

2. Drugs:

A common essential part of managing interstitial cystitis is medical intervention.

• Painkillers:

• Prescription drugs or over-the-counter painkillers may be used to treat IC-related pain.

• Installations of Bladders:

• To treat inflammation and ease symptoms, medications such as dimethyl sulfoxide (DMSO) may be injected directly into the bladder.

• Oral Drugs:

• Certain drugs, such as pentosan polysulfate sodium (Elmiron), may be recommended in order to aid with bladder lining healing.

• Mast cell stabilizers and antihistamines:

• These drugs may be used to lower inflammation and regulate the immune system.

3. Changes In Lifestyle:

Modifications to one's lifestyle may help control symptoms and improve general health.

• Training for Bladders:

Increasing the intervals between toilet trips and scheduling voiding may both assist with bladder function.

• Managing Fluids:

• It might be helpful to stay well hydrated while limiting excess consumption, particularly of chemicals that irritate the bladder.

• Consistent Exercise:

• Regular, gentle exercise may improve general health and perhaps lessen the symptoms of IC.

• Giving Up Smoking:

• Smoking might make IC symptoms worse; giving it up may help symptoms get better.

4. Alternative Medical Interventions:

• Acupuncture:

• Acupuncture, which includes inserting tiny needles into certain body sites, helps some people with IC symptoms.

• Supplements with herbs:

• The possible anti-inflammatory benefits of certain herbal supplements, including quercetin or supplements comprising a blend of herbs, may be investigated.

• Body-Mind Methods:

• Mind-body methods like yoga and biofeedback may help control the symptoms of IC by lowering stress and encouraging relaxation.

• Nutritional Supplements:

• As part of an all-encompassing treatment approach, omega-3 fatty acids and other supplements with anti-inflammatory qualities may be taken into consideration.

It's crucial to remember that each person will respond differently to these therapies, and a customized strategy is often required. Speaking with a medical expert, such as a pelvic pain specialist or urologist, is essential to creating a customized treatment plan that takes into account each patient's unique requirements and symptoms. Furthermore, it is crucial to maintain constant contact with medical professionals in order to track development and modify the treatment plan as necessary.

CHAPTER SIX
Nutritional Techniques

Urinary urgency and frequency are the hallmarks of Interstitial Cystitis (IC), a chronic illness sometimes referred to as painful bladder syndrome.

Although the precise origin of IC is unknown, research points to a major influence that nutrition may have in symptom management and quality of life enhancement for those who have the condition. This is a thorough examination of the idea of dietary approaches to the treatment of interstitial cystitis:

The Function Of Food In The Treatment Of Interstitial Cystitis:

1. Irritation and Inflammation:

• Bladder lining irritation and inflammation are often linked to IC. Some meals have the potential to worsen these symptoms, making them more painful and uncomfortable.

• An anti-inflammatory and anti-irritating diet is essential for controlling the symptoms of IC.

2. Eliminating Trigger Foods:

• Foods High in Acid:

• The acids in citrus fruits, tomatoes, and their byproducts might irritate the lining of the bladder. Limiting or avoiding these is advised.

• Spicy Foods:

• For some people, spices and spicy peppers might exacerbate their symptoms. It is best to cut them down or remove them entirely from the diet.

• Coffee:

• Caffeine is known to irritate the bladder and might make it seem more urgent and frequent. This covers tea, coffee, chocolate, and a few soft drinks.

• Constructed Sweeteners:

• Aspartame and saccharin are two sweets that might make IC symptoms worse. It could be wiser to use natural sweeteners like maple syrup or honey instead.

• Alcohol:

• Because alcohol may irritate the bladder, people with IC should minimize or stay away from it.

• Foods with a lot of processing:

• Preservatives and chemicals used in processed foods can cause inflammation. A diet high in whole foods and low in processed foods is usually advised.

3. Nutritional Assistance for Healthy Bladder:

• Hydration:

• Staying well hydrated is essential for good health and may help dilute urine, which lessens the possibility of irritation.

• Fatty Acids Omega-3:

• Foods high in omega-3 fatty acids, such as walnuts, flaxseeds, and fatty fish (salmon, mackerel), may reduce inflammation and promote bladder health.

• Foods High in Quercetin:

• A naturally occurring antioxidant with possible anti-inflammatory effects is quercetin. Good sources include foods like kale, apples, and berries.

• Prebiotics:

• Yogurt and fermented foods include probiotics, which may help maintain a balanced population of gut bacteria and hence lower levels of inflammation in general.

Tailored Food Programs:

1. Meal Journal:

• Maintaining a thorough food journal assists in pinpointing unique triggers for every person. This might help in formulating a customized nutrition plan.

2. Gradual Removal:

• A progressive reduction of possible trigger foods enables a deeper knowledge of the effects of each food item rather than a dramatic overhaul.

3. Meeting with a Nutritionist:

• It might be very helpful to work with a qualified dietician who has knowledge of managing IC. They may assist in avoiding triggers and assisting in the creation of a diet that is both nutritionally sufficient and balanced.

4. Trial and Error:

• People may need to try changing their diet by reintroducing things one at a time that they were told to avoid and seeing how that worked. This aids in optimizing the customized eating schedule.

In summary, nutritional approaches are essential for the treatment of interstitial cystitis. For those with IC, implementing a customized diet plan that emphasizes lowering inflammation, staying away from trigger foods, and promoting bladder health can greatly help with symptom management and quality of life enhancement. Always seek the advice of medical professionals for individualized guidance based on specific needs and conditions.

CHAPTER SEVEN

Interstitial Cystitis Coping Mechanisms:

Urinary urgency and frequency are the hallmarks of Interstitial Cystitis (IC), a chronic illness sometimes referred to as painful bladder syndrome. The emotional tolls that IC can have on people as well as its physical symptoms are addressed in a comprehensive coping strategy. This is a comprehensive guide to coping mechanisms that emphasizes mental and emotional health, managing chronic pain, creating a network of support, and using mind-body methods:

1. Mental And Emotional Health:

a. Acceptance and Mindfulness: - Recognize that having IC is a reality and use mindfulness to be in the moment. - Mindfulness meditation can enhance general mental health and assist in stress management.

b. Therapeutic Support: - To address the psychological effects of IC, take into consideration therapy options like cognitive-behavioral therapy (CBT). - Counseling can help with coping strategies and transitioning to new lifestyles.

c. Education: Learn about IC to have a better understanding of the illness. Having knowledge enables people to make well-informed choices about their health.

d. Journaling: - Record your feelings, triggers, and symptoms in a diary. This may reveal trends and provide guidance on practical coping mechanisms.

2. Handling Prolonged Pain:

a. Pain Management Techniques: - Create a customized pain management strategy in collaboration with medical specialists. Examine your alternatives for medication, physical therapy, and complementary treatments such as acupuncture.

b. Heat and Cold Therapy: Depending on the location afflicted, either heat or cold may help reduce pain and suffering.

c. Gentle Exercise: To keep up your physical activity level without aggravating your symptoms, try low-impact activities like yoga, swimming, or strolling.

d. Activity pacing is important to prevent overexertion, which may exacerbate IC symptoms.

3. Putting Together A Support Network:

a. Openly discuss IC with friends, family, and coworkers in order to promote tolerance and support. - Educate your support network on your requirements and limits.

b. Join Support Groups: - Connect with others who have IC via support groups, both online and offline. - Sharing experiences and advice may offer a sense of community and lessen feelings of loneliness.

c. Family Involvement: - Encourage family members to engage in educational sessions to better appreciate the problems and modifications required.

4. Mind-Body Methodologies:

a. Relaxation Techniques: - Practice deep breathing techniques and gradual muscular relaxation to control stress and improve relaxation.

b. Biofeedback: - Explore biofeedback treatment to acquire control over automatic biological processes, perhaps lowering pain and discomfort.

c. Yoga and Meditation: - Incorporate mild yoga and meditation into your regimen to enhance physical and mental well-being.

d. hypnosis: - Some people find relief with hypnosis, which may assist in controlling pain perception and enhance overall comfort.

In conclusion, managing interstitial cystitis involves a comprehensive strategy that addresses physical symptoms, mental well-being, and the creation of a strong support system. By combining medicinal therapies with lifestyle improvements and psychological support, persons with IC may increase their quality of life and better manage the problems associated with this chronic illness.

CHAPTER EIGHT
Living With Interstitial Cystitis

Living with Interstitial Cystitis (IC) may be tough, but with correct care and lifestyle adaptations, people can have satisfying lives. Interstitial Cystitis is a chronic ailment characterized by bladder discomfort, urgency, and frequency, and it typically needs a multidisciplinary strategy to manage its effect on everyday living. Here's a thorough discussion of the ideas you've mentioned:

Tips For Daily Life:
Dietary Adjustments:

Recognize and stay away from items that may act as triggers for IC symptoms, such as coffee, acidic meals, spicy foods, and artificial sweeteners.

Keep a food journal to monitor your own triggers and trends.

Drinking plenty of water

Hydrate yourself with plenty of water; dehydration exacerbates the symptoms of IC. But avoid bladder irritants and drink water instead of other liquids.

Urinary Health:

Exercise your pelvic floor to build up the muscles that support your bladder.

Maintain a regular schedule for voiding to avoid the bladder filling up too much, which will lessen the chance of flare-ups.

Handling Stress:

Since stress may make IC worse, try stress-relieving practices like yoga, meditation, or deep breathing techniques to help control symptoms.

Pain Control:

Consult with medical specialists about pain management techniques, which may include prescription drugs, physical therapy, or complementary treatments like acupuncture.

Handling Social And Professional Activities:

Interaction:

Inform coworkers and employers in an honest manner about your illness, including any possible obstacles and any modifications that could be required.

Workplace Perquisites:

To successfully manage symptoms, ask for accommodations like comfortable chairs, flexible work hours, or pauses for bathroom breaks.

Taking Care of Oneself at Work:

Establish a cozy workstation that takes ergonomics into account, and carry the supplies you'll need (like heated pads) to covertly manage your symptoms.

Social Assistance:

Create a network of support among coworkers and friends at work and in social settings by teaching them about IC to promote empathy and understanding.

When Carrying Interstitial Cystitis:

Getting ready:

Make sure to properly plan your travels, considering the closeness and availability of restrooms.

For extended travels, include necessities like a heating pad, prescription drugs, and cozy clothes.

Accessibility of restrooms:

When planning a trip, look into the availability of bathrooms in the area and think about using applications that provide this information.

Staying Hydrated While on the Go:

When traveling, remember to stay hydrated and to be mindful of any possible triggers.

Partnerships And Closeness:

Interaction with the Partner:

Discuss openly with your spouse the signs and symptoms of IC, as well as triggers and ways that they can help you.

Management of Intimacy:

Try different poses and activities to see what makes you feel the least uncomfortable during intimacy.

Plan your alone time for when your symptoms are at their lowest.

Psychological Assistance:

Since IC may affect mental health, consider attending support groups or couples therapy to address the emotional component of dealing with the illness.

Compassion & Forbearance:

Encourage tolerance and understanding in relationships since IC flare-ups often necessitate adjusting schedules and activities. IC can be unexpected.

In conclusion, self-care routines, honest communication, and lifestyle modifications are all necessary for living with interstitial cystitis. With the correct techniques, people with IC may travel, work, socialize, and sustain deep relationships while still successfully managing their symptoms. Personalized advice from healthcare specialists is essential when creating a management strategy that will work and last.

CHAPTER NINE
Upcoming Perspectives

Painful bladder syndrome, another name for interstitial cystitis (IC), is a persistent illness that causes pain or discomfort in the bladder and surrounding pelvic area. Although there is currently no known treatment for IC, patient advocacy initiatives, new treatments, and continuing research provide patients who have the illness hope for better care and a higher quality of life.

Upcoming Horizons

1. More Advanced Diagnostic Instruments:

Future developments could bring forth more precise and effective diagnostic instruments. This may include identifying certain indicators linked to IC via genetic testing, enhanced imaging methods, or biomarkers.

2. Personalized Health Care:

• A move in the direction of individualized medicine may be coming for IC therapy in the future. More efficient and focused treatments may result from customizing treatment regimens according to each patient's unique symptoms, genetic composition, and therapy response.

3. Digital Health Solutions:

• As digital health gains popularity, wearable technology and applications that let people track symptoms, keep an eye on triggers, and instantly connect with medical professionals may be part of the solutions of the future. This may provide useful information for physicians and patients alike.

Novel Research And Treatments:

1. Research on Microbiomes:

• Studies on the function of the microbiota in IC are still ongoing. Gaining insight into how the microbiota of the bladder and the stomach interact may lead to the development of novel therapeutic approaches, such as probiotics or therapies that modify the microbiome.

2. Immunotherapy:

• The goal of emerging treatments for IC may be to alter the immunological response. Investigations are being conducted on immunomodulatory medications and treatments that target the inflammatory pathways connected to IC.

3. Methods Based on Neurology:

• Because IC has neurological components, research into medicines that target the nervous system is continuing. Techniques for neuromodulation, such as sacral nerve stimulation, are being investigated for their potential to treat symptoms of inflammatory constipation.

Treatment Strategies That Look Good:

1. Bladder Instability:

• The use of drugs such as lidocaine or heparin for bladder instillations shows promise in relieving symptoms. To improve the composition and delivery strategies for these injections, research is continuously being conducted.

2. Dietary Adjustments:

• New research indicates that dietary modifications, such as removing certain foods and drinks, may have an effect on the symptoms of IC. Dietary advice for the management of IC may be improved and expanded by future studies.

3. Stem Cell Utilization:

• The use of stem cells in treatment to treat damaged bladder tissue is now being investigated. While preliminary research seems encouraging, further studies are required to confirm the product's safety and effectiveness.

Patient Advocacy And Involvement In The Community:

1. Increasing Conscience

• Patient advocacy organizations are essential in spreading knowledge about intractable constipation. Raising awareness may result in better comprehension of the illness among the general public and medical experts, as well as earlier diagnosis and less stigma.

2. Funding for Research:

The main goal of advocacy work is to get money for IC research. More funding may spur research projects, improving our knowledge of the illness and paving the way for the creation of more potent remedies.

3. Patient Support and Education:

• Advocacy organizations play a crucial role in offering IC sufferers support groups and educational materials. Giving patients more information about their illnesses might help them take better care of themselves and be in better overall health.

In summary, new treatments, continued research, and patient advocates' active participation all point to a promising future for the management of interstitial cystitis. It is anticipated that as these several facets develop further, the group's endeavor to comprehend, manage, and assist people suffering from IC will significantly improve the lives of those impacted by this difficult illness.

Conclusion

In summary, treating Interstitial Cystitis (IC) requires a multifaceted, holistic approach that takes social, psychological, and physical factors into account. There have been many obstacles to overcome and a great deal of advancement made in the understanding and management of IC. The intricacy of this illness necessitates a streamlined strategy for treatment that stresses education and support-based empowerment in addition to medical therapies.

Taking Stock Of The Trip:

The quest to comprehend and manage interstitial cystitis has been characterized by an ongoing investigation of the many elements that contribute to the illness. Researchers and medical experts have studied the intricacies of IC throughout time, revealing its complicated nature. The medical community has shown remarkable resilience in the face of an illness that severely affects the quality of life for a great number of people. This resilience has been shown throughout the journey, from the early difficulties in identifying the ailment to the current research aimed at revealing its underlying causes.

Acknowledging the advancements in diagnostic criteria refinement that have made it possible to identify IC patients more precisely is essential. A deeper knowledge of IC has been made possible by developments in medical imaging, biomarker discovery, and the role inflammation plays in the illness. By thinking back on this trip, we can recognize the cooperative efforts of patients, doctors, and researchers who are all trying to solve the puzzle of IC.

Advances In The Knowledge Of Interstitial Cystitis:

Advances in our knowledge of IC have improved our ability to diagnose patients and opened the door to more specialized and efficient treatment plans. A more individualized approach to care has been made possible by the discovery of subtypes within IC, acknowledging that every person's experience with IC may be unique. The expanding knowledge of IC has created opportunities for innovative therapeutic approaches, from the recognition of the bladder epithelium's function to the investigation of neurogenic and inflammatory components.

Furthermore, improvements in patient-reported outcome measures and the inclusion of patient viewpoints in research have made it possible to gain a deeper understanding of how IC affects people's lives. In addition to improving research results, this patient-centered approach has given people with IC the confidence to actively engage in their healthcare decisions.

Providing Information And Assistance To Empower People:

Providing medical care alone is not enough to empower people with IC; a comprehensive support network that takes into account the social, psychological, and emotional aspects of living with a chronic illness is also necessary. During this journey, knowledge becomes a potent tool that empowers people to take an active role in their own self-care, make educated decisions about their treatment options, and gain a better understanding of their condition.

Among people impacted by IC, support groups and educational materials are essential for establishing a sense of community. Peer support can be a powerful tool for people, providing them with the chance to exchange life experiences, coping mechanisms, and insightful opinions. Furthermore, through encouraging open communication, giving patients easily understandable information, and involving patients in joint decision-making, healthcare providers significantly contribute to patients' empowerment.

In summary, a comprehensive and patient-centered approach that takes into account the experiences of those impacted by IC is necessary in addition to medical interventions for a simplified solution approach.

Understanding IC better and enabling people with information and assistance creates the groundwork for a more humane and efficient approach to treating this difficult illness. As time goes on, expanding our knowledge and enhancing the quality of life for people with interstitial cystitis will require sustained cooperation between researchers, medical professionals, and patients.

THE END

www.ingramcontent.com/pod-product-compliance
Lightning Source LLC
Chambersburg PA
CBHW050748260726